I0420788

Sunshine Vitamin
& Black People

Sunshine Vitamin & Black People

THE POWER OF VITAMIN D

Jay Parker

Jay Parker, Copyright C 2015
ALL RIGHTS RESERVED
The author is hereby established as the sole holder of the copyright.

ISBN: 1519334729
ISBN 13: 9781519334725

Content

About the Author

Jay Parker believes that each choice you make regarding your food and vitamin D lifestyle acts as either a deposit into or withdrawal from your "health banking" account. You can choose to make mostly savings deposits or check withdrawals. The balance of that account determines your energy, vitality, risk of disease, longevity, and ultimately the quality of your life.

Jay Parker has worked in big food companies creating concepts. Jay Parker, fondly referred to as J.P., writes to inspire a healthy relationship with food and exercise, along with practical tips to incorporate healthy living. And yes, he was a bartender at a point in time.

Preface

Vitamin D is a superstar vitamin. Try imagining plants. Plants blossom under the Sun. Photosynthesis takes place under the Sun.

Humans do photosynthesis too under the sun. Human skin does the process. Without the Sun, plants get sick. Without the Sun, human skin cannot make vitamin D easily and cheaply.

Vitamin D plays many roles in the body, including modulation of cell growth, neuromuscular and immune function, and reduction of inflammation among many other roles.

As important as vitamin D is, there are people who are uninformed about the deadly results of vitamin D deficiency. There are those who have the luxury of 366-day sunshine. In such climates, no thought is giving as to adequate intake -- the optimal level of vitamin D.

This is because the people are out in the Sun daily. They are black people. They enjoy the benefits of the Sun until they emigrate to USA, UK, Australia, Europe etc.

In their new abode, they will start to suffer osteoporosis, various cancers and other debilitating cold weather illnesses. They forfeited some of the Sun's benefits because some of them refuse to sunbathe anymore as they want to be light skinned.

Approximately 40 million adults in the United States have osteoporosis. Many are at risk of developing osteoporosis, a disease characterized by low bone mass and structural deterioration of bone tissue that increases the chances for bones to be fragile and so increases the risk of bone fractures.

Osteoporosis is mostly associated with inadequate calcium intakes. Deficiency in vitamin D contributes to osteoporosis by reducing calcium absorption. And the most people identified in cold climates with vitamin D deficiency are black peoples.

Let us not forget that optimal levels of vitamin D enables you to burn fat so that you do not have a buildup in your buttocks, thighs and belly.

CHAPTER 1

Introduction

Everyone has something that makes them unique. Every nation has its uniqueness in the way and manner they receive the sunlight. Ok, that should be whether the clime is equatorial or not and whether the climate is ice cold or hot. Every race has something that makes them unique. For this topic, it is mostly in your skin color.

The black skin has its uniqueness. That uniqueness, is through the Sun where the sunshine vitamin, a vitamin that we like to nickname the black vitamin.

When you walk through the park in the summer you see some sunbathers. Which race of peoples do you observe sunbathing?

I don't know about you but I always observe white folks. I hardly see Chinese and other Asians, Africans and or Hispanics.

Ordinarily, the people you should see should be black skinned people because they need the intense sunlight most. Black skin is a marvel. It is black for a reason. It evolved to be black so as to be able tap into the Sun and get those properties that will give you long life, full of health, stronger and biologically efficient.

To tell you how biologically efficient black people are, I will let you in on how much black people were priced by the rich landowners of the slave era. A black slave was valued at seventy five British pounds while a white Irish slave fetched five British pounds.

The white skin needs the Sun but not that much. More than fifteen minutes in the Sun without sunscreen and they will get burns and ultimately peels. Black folks need it far more and they don't get scorched in fifteen minutes even without sunscreen.

It is that vitamin known as a pre-vitamin D when processed and assimilated as vitamin D3. If you lose that which makes you unique, you lose that which gave you those characteristics of blackness and dominance in sports and in health.

Black skin is unique. It is unique because nature made black people unique. This is a health talk not pandering. Biblical Adam is black. Eve is black.

The Jews were black. Ask Ethiopian sons of Solomon. Solomon's Ethiopian children were true royals. They still are.

Blackness is the reason black people suffer very little (until recently) of cancer, multiple sclerosis, and those other cold weather afflictions. I feel for people living out of the equator but, they have learned to know better the science of vitamin D. Those blacks living outside the equator must also comprehend the science of vitamin D in cold climes.

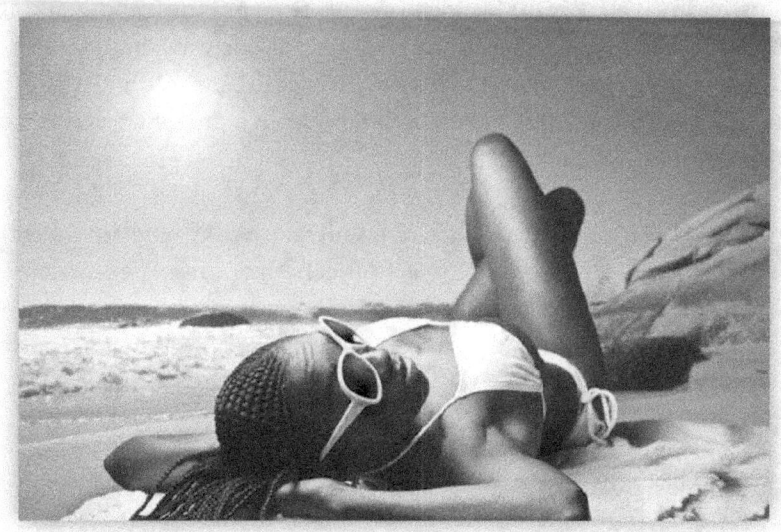

Sunbathing

While the white people are seeking ways to absorb more of the black vitamins, black folks in diaspora are dodging the Sun.

Why is this happening? Easy answer. Forget science for a minute. We will come to that in subsequent chapters. For now, let us follow the ancestors of the African Americans.

Africans in Africa continues to bake in the sun. They cannot avoid it. The few that can afford to avoid the Sun (the rich ones) have been afflicted with different types of cancer and unexplainable deaths. Any wonder then, when you read the obituaries of rich Africans, you read stuff on the lines of "died of unknown causes". I am used to thinking that unknown meant hidden inexplicable disease.

Obviously, they knew not the afflictions. They knew not because their source of information—the white man is yet to really understand the Sun.

The Sun is black man's big friend and white man's little friend. You could believe it, like it, hate it, love it, and research it all you want, but for millions of years, the black skin (not just black man) have experienced and lived it for that long. For the black skin, the sunshine vitamin is priceless. It is the black man's Vitamin. The Sun.

Lots of African Americans and immigrant blacks tend to avoid the Sun if they could. Yet, the Sun made African Americans. The Sun defined them. The Sun made them black. The Sun said, here I am, I am your God. I, defined you. Without me, you are no longer black. I AM in you and you in me.

But some Africans and other diaspora Africans hate the Sun.

They cannot wait to explain. Some have even tried to change the structure of their skin. They buy creams. They buy creams that can change black skin to lighter color. Creams that can change black to white. None can change white to black though. These lightening creams are manufactured by white people's businesses for black people's use. The manufacture of lightening creams is an indication that the manufacturers hardly understand the working of sunlight on skin. It is also an indication that the users of lightening creams hardly understand the damage they are causing to their black skin.

Is it not ironic that while some black folks are lightening up, some white folks are darkening down? They call it tanning and it does not come cheap either. If it were possible to inject melanin, some folks will give it a try. Unless, a way of injecting melanin safely into the white skin is discovered, tanning will continue to thrive.

White folks have convinced majority in the world into thinking that the white skin is the norm. It is not. In the land of skin colors, people with lily white skin succumb to diseases faster than most. Naturally, white skin is defective under the Sun so to speak.

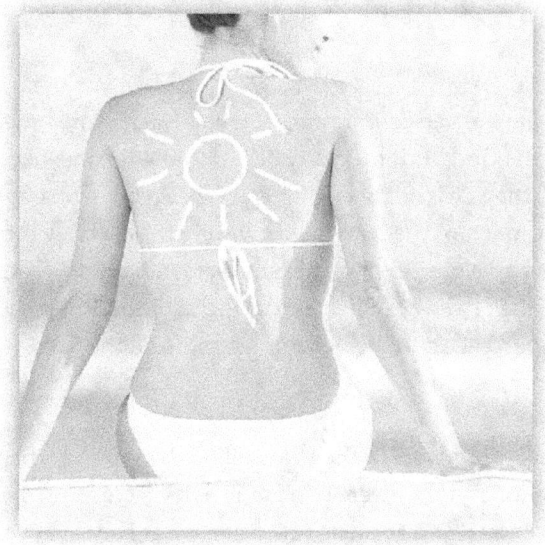

In the above picture: what do you think will happen to that
skin if it stays sunbathing for more than one hour?

Most people have been conditioned to think that white skin is better. That is far from the truth. Black folks are most guilty of this. They have been so ridiculously conditioned to think white skin is better.

In the days of slavery, the rich land owners valued the dark skin. They valued Africans 70 British pounds more than the 5 British pounds they paid for the white slaves.

White people planted the divide and rule tactics of color. And perhaps, white skin was not the original. They were not the originals. They balk at the Sun. They cannot stay too long in the Sun. The Sun gives them sunburn.

Yes, because the Sun is "black" so to speak. The Sun is life for the black skin. The Sun is why the earth has life. The Sun was at a point in history deified as God. But no more.

Africans in diaspora have lost their bearings for white man's lifestyle and thoughts. Oh boy. It is terrible. What do you expect when you dump your "Sun God"-- you end up getting cancer, multiple sclerosis and many others?

Blacks who are versed in history know how our forefathers talked and represented the Gods. It is their way of explaining the inexplicable. In some African tales, the Sun is not taking for granted. Egyptian pharaoh Akhenaten, thought that much of the Sun. He knew something about the Sun. To him, the Sun was marvelous. To him, the Sun was symbolically, God. If only black folks thought half the way Akhenaten thought, of the Sun. Akhenaten recognized the importance and the benefits we get from the Sun.

Your forefathers were in the fields tilling the ground. That is what they were created for and they were good at it. They were in the Sun toiling and getting rejuvenated and re-engineered skin wise. The skin evolved because of the Sun's intense sunlight. The black skin's ability to make optimal level of vitamin D, is reason why you are biologically superior. Enjoy your superiority to your heart's desire if you understand how to tap into the Sun's energy. The way to attain optimal level of vitamin D is what this work is all about.

Vitamin D is getting a lot of attention lately even in medical circles. Many people are having their vitamin D levels tested and are surprised to find out that they are low in this essential hormone.

What exactly is Vitamin D and why should you care about your Vitamin D levels? How does sunscreen use, contribute to deficiency in this important vitamin, and what can we do to remedy the deficiency?

This book has been written in such a way that you will be able to absorb the contents in less than it takes to travel from one point to another in a bus or train ride.

Vitamin D is actually not a vitamin. It is a hormone. A very essential hormone. If you are deficient in this hormone, you will literally fall apart. You will be shocked how deficient, people are of this vitamin. It is a beautiful thing, every day in equatorial Africa and an apt description for that matter, to consider that every day is a full day of free Vitamin D.

For Africans, every day is in a season the white folk calls summer. If you understand why there are dark and white skin people you will understand why there are a diversity of skin colors in the world. They come in varying colors. You will then understand how our various skin color connects us to our evolution or adaptation to our environments.

Vitamin D is produced from exposure to sunlight. Call it human photo-synthesis if you wish. UV light from the Sun starts off a chemical reaction in our skin to produce the precursor to Vitamin D. With help from the liver and kidneys, the chemical reaction started in the skin turns into active Vitamin D3 that our bodies can use.

The Sun gives health to humans and animals like it gives plants life. You better think of this seriously. If you think about how the Sun gives humans the sunshine health, you will not be running out of Sun with excuses like "it will make me darker" and some other excuses such as it burns and it peels the skin.

Most of us will remember learning in elementary school about photo-synthesis-- the study of how plants capture the light of the sun and turn it into energy. Some might even still remember how to write the chemical equation too.

What we were not told by our teachers then was that humans actually do similar photosynthesis to create vitamin D. Africa, the continent, has an abundance of the health giving equatorial sun rays.

She has been enjoying this hormone in the form of natural vitamin D from time. That is why the black skin has evolved so as to get more of the nourishing natural sunshine vitamin.

No dosages, No prescriptions.

People of African descent are fortunate to have less visible signs of aging such as wrinkles, fine lines and age spots as compared to some other variations of skin colors. Africans in the equator are even more fortunate and privileged. This is due to the high amount of melanin produced by their skin. Melanin gives color to the skin, eyes, and hair. And there is a reason why the color of the black people is the way it is. The eyes can tolerate more direct sunlight without sun blocking glasses.

The more melanin you have, the darker your skin. The more you take the sunlight, the more you accumulate the joys of good health associated with vitamin D.

People of African descent, living in cold climate, can have a natural Sun protection factor (SPF) of up to 13 as compared to 3-4 for whites. For equatorial and other hot weather blacks, it is even better. This advantage for African Americans and black immigrants, can also be a disadvantage. It is a double edged sword for black people not living in equatorial climate. You just need to have proper information with which to turn the disadvantage into an advantage.

Now, they (those who deal with skin and those who deal with hormones) are telling Africans that the sunlight causes cancer. And Africans fell for it. What group of Africans did they carry out research on? Did any school in Gabon, Ghana or South Africa do any investigating?

Of course we know how the research thing goes. White professionals do the investigative studies perhaps using white skin persons. The results are then published and accepted for the whole world including black skin people. It is not just simply insane, it is presumptuous.

And much of Africa depends on the west for its medical information. They discard old practices which have kept them alive when western medicine was not available.

Thus, the dark African skin awaits studies done on white skin to apply to Africans when it should be the other way round. That way is to study black skins, publish the findings and let the people accept or reject the benefits if any.

Studies now show that most black people who travel out of Africa are most likely to be deficient in vitamin D. It is so because the privilege of free equatorial sunlight is no longer a privilege. Black immigrants just take vitamin D for granted like Africans do in Africa. In Africa, all you need do is take a fifteen to thirty-minute walk--depending on the time of day and weather-- to a friend's house and your body makes all the Vitamin D it needs for the day and some extra to spare.

Unfortunately, dermatologists tell white folks that direct sun rays is bad for their skin. Yep. White skin, they said. And voila, everyone, including black folks queued up. As they queued for the white man's dermatologist information, they started to lose the health they enjoyed for free from time. I know a man who is in his late 90s. He lives in equatorial Africa. He has his complete original teeth- thirty two of them.

People of less than fifty years old in United States and other temperate zones may have had half their teeth pulled. And we have many good dentists too here in the United States and temperate places. The rate of cancer is up among black folks too.

CHAPTER 2
Statistics from CDC

See some stats from CDC

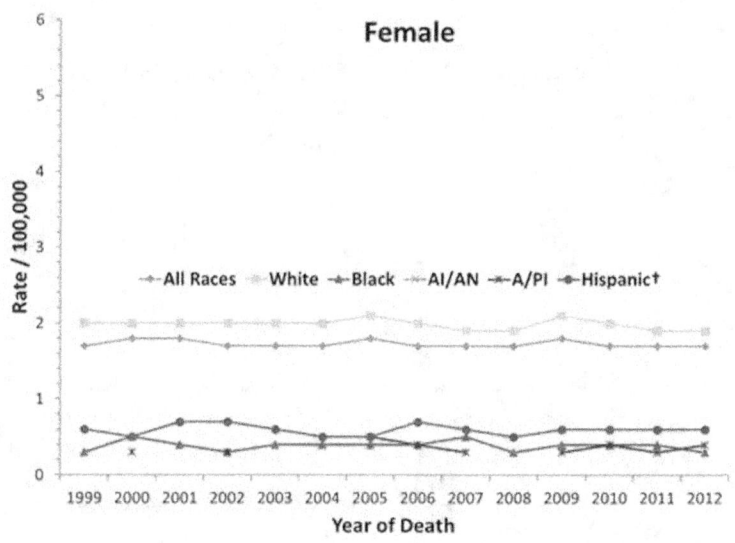

The rate of people getting melanoma of the skin or dying from melanoma of the skin varies by race and ethnicity.

Incidence Rates by Race/Ethnicity

"Incidence rate" means how many people out of a given number get the disease each year. The graph below shows how many people out of 100,000 got melanoma of the skin each year during the years 1999–2012. The year 2012 is the most recent year for which numbers have been reported. The melanoma of the skin incidence rate is grouped by race and ethnicity.

The graph below shows that in 2012, among men, white men had the highest rate of getting melanoma of the skin, followed by American Indian/Alaska Native, Hispanic, Asian/Pacific Islander, and black men. Among women, white women had the highest rate of getting melanoma of the skin, followed by American Indian/Alaska Native, Hispanic, Asian/Pacific Islander, and black women.

Skin Cancer
Incidence Rates* by Race and Ethnicity, U.S., 1999–2012

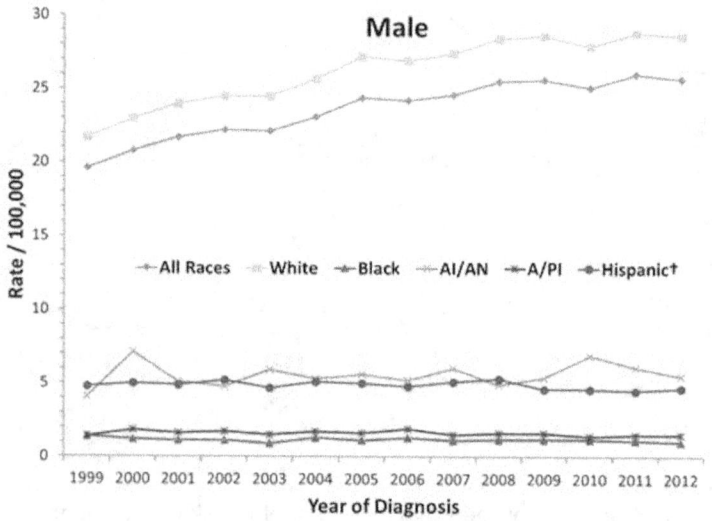

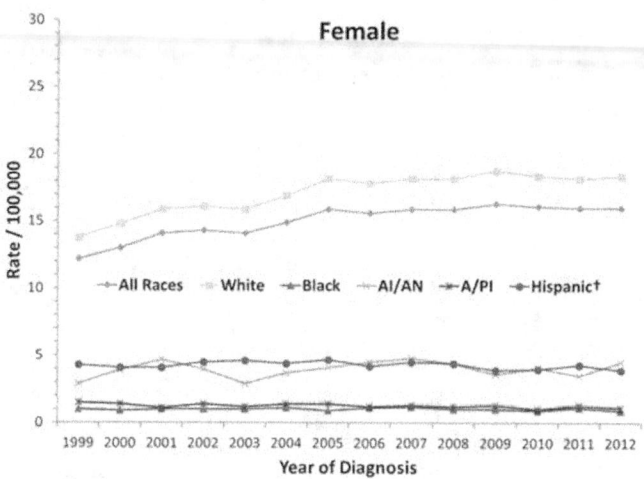

Incidence source: Combined data from the National Program of Cancer Registries as submitted to CDC and from the Surveillance, Epidemiology and End Results program as submitted to the National Cancer Institute in November 2014.

*Rates are per 100,000 and are age-adjusted to the 2000 U.S. standard population (19 age groups – Census P25-1130). Incidence rates are for state registries that meet USCS publication criteria for all years, 1999–2012. Incidence rates cover about 92% of the U.S. population.

†Hispanic origin is not mutually exclusive from race categories (white, black, Asian/Pacific Islander, American Indian/Alaska Native).

Death Rates by Race/Ethnicity

From 1999–2012, the rate of people dying from melanoma of the skin varies. It depends on their race and ethnicity. Here is a graph below which shows that in 2012, among men, white men were more likely to die of melanoma of the skin than any other group. They are followed by Hispanic then black and Asian/Pacific Islander men. Among women, again, white women were more likely to die of melanoma of the skin than any other group, followed by Hispanic, Asian/Pacific Islander, and black women.

Skin Cancer
Death Rates* by Race and Ethnicity, U.S., 1999–2012

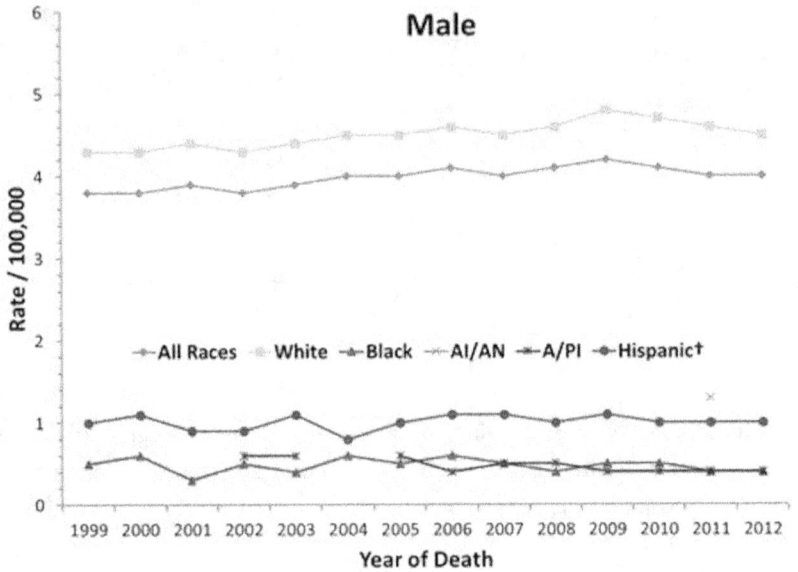

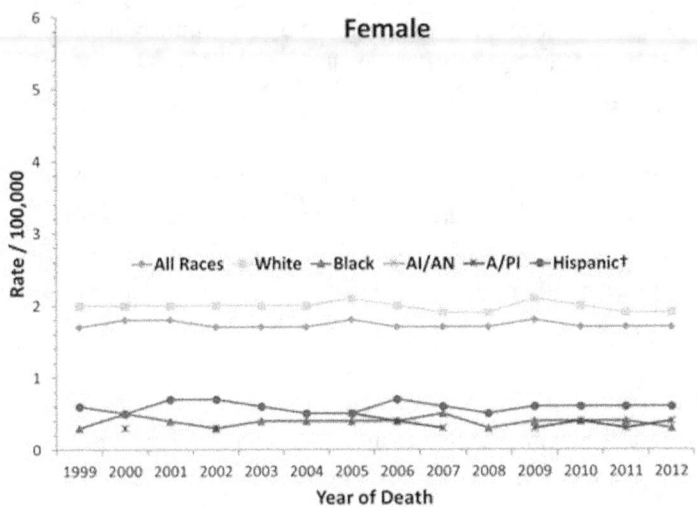

The way it is, it will take years to correct the impression and damage that both endocrinologists and dermatologists have done educating the masses, black skinned people included -- that the sun is dangerous to the skin- all skin types. That is the impression then and that is the impression now.

That impression is out there even though that is not the whole truth.

The truth is, that black skin evolved while white skin adapted to a climate with less intense sunlight.

Endocrinologists did not fare any better in informing black folks either. Endocrinologists - those that treat people who suffer from hormonal imbalances, typically from glands in the endocrine system.

The overall goal of treatment is to restore the normal balance of hormones found in a patient's body. They failed to challenge and dispute the information put on the table by dermatologists.

They should have lectured us all about the important hormones the sunshine produces. Does this sound like some form of ignorance? Some could say—yes, it is.

But remember, their studies were done for the health of white skin. It is therefore safe to say that there is a lot of ignorance within the black community. Not everyone is well informed about the effects of vitamin D deficiency. From those who are informed, the information cannot "trickle down" to patients fast enough.

Much of Africa is inside or very close to the equator, allowing its human, animal and plant inhabitants get intense year-round sun exposure, intense enough to stimulate vitamin D production in dark-skinned Africans. Because of this intense year-round sun exposure, Africans evolved to have dark skin to bring about to the barest minimum the effects of vitamin D deficiency.

The skin color evolved in the African environment to strike a balance between fulfilling their vitamin D needs and protecting themselves from overexposure to the Sun.

According to some published studies (studies likely done on white skin) elderly adults who were moderately deficient in vitamin D has a 53% increased risk of developing dementia. That same risk skyrockets to 125% in those who were severely deficient. The same results were also shown for Alzheimer's patients.

These are obviously very scary results, but so are the possible outcomes of Sun damage to white skin. Sun is the key ingredient for the only vitamin that we can make ourselves-vitamin D.

Another sickness to reminisce about is multiple sclerosis. That should give you a reason to start getting your daily requirement of vitamin D.

Multiple sclerosis is more common in certain geographical areas of the world, particularly areas that are farther from the equator. Prevalence is generally highest in European and North American cities and countries.

The clustering of multiple sclerosis cases in these regions has led researchers to investigate whether certain toxins, infections, or vitamin deficiencies (such as vitamin D) may play a factor in triggering multiple sclerosis in genetically susceptible people.

The truth of the matter is that no matter how you dice the results, multiple sclerosis is not rampant in equatorial Africa where the supply of the sunshine vitamin is readily and naturally abundant.

However, there is a study done by Kaiser Permanente. According to this study which was published in Neurology- a journal-- multiple sclerosis is more common in black women in Southern California--United States. This study must make you wonder especially if you are of the black race because this finding runs contrary to generally peddled belief that the incidence of multiple sclerosis is generally less in the black communities.

The report concludes that black patients had a 47 percent higher risk of MS than white patients. Hispanics and Asians had a 50 percent and 80 percent lower risks compared to white patients respectively.

Thus the conclusion was "Our findings do not support the widely accepted assertion that blacks have a lower risk of MS than whites. A possible explanation for our findings is that people with darker skin tones have lower vitamin D levels and thereby an increased risk of MS, but this would not explain why Hispanics and Asians have a lower risk of MS than whites or why the higher risk of MS among blacks was found only among women".

Before you rush to accept these findings, let us ponder over these questions

1. How many of these dark skin persons especially women bathed in the sun as required? Africans in the equator has the lowest incidence of MS. Why is that so?
2. Darker varied skins' requires stronger UV rays-- did these women whose files were looked at even take a 15 minutes sun bath?
3. What was their daily supplement intake of vitamin D if any?

Something to bear in mind is that it takes less time for white skin to make all the vitamin D it needs. White skin has less protection from the Sun. It takes more time for the black skin to make the same amount of vitamin D because black skin has protections from the sunlight. Until all African Americans and black immigrants understand this, it will get worse.

Geographical variation in the prevalence of multiple sclerosis is striking. Multiple sclerosis is rare in equatorial countries--sunny hot countries. Most studies have come to the finding that multiple sclerosis is common as you move away from the equator. The variation is well pronounced in Northern European cities and peoples, especially those with Scandinavian ancestry in affected populations. African Americans are no longer as safe from this disease as they once believed.

All in all there is also an environmental influence. Some studies in the United States have northern areas with a prevalence of over 100 per 100,000 and only 20 per 100,000 in southern states. Simply put, you get more Sun in the south. The chances that you will bake in the Sun is higher if you lived in the south.

That multiple sclerosis is more common in black women than in white women, according to that Kaiser Permanente study published in the journal Neurology must make any black skinned person living in North America stop and ask themselves those questions that were asked earlier with regards to the sufficiency or deficiency of their daily intake of vitamin D since the findings run contrary to the widely accepted belief that blacks are less susceptible to MS, according to the researchers.

Let us repeat. That blacks who live in North America and indeed blacks who run away from the rays of the Sun are more likely to suffer the bad consequences of vitamin D deficiency.

Simply do not be vitamin D'fficient.

Stop now and think for a minute. Be honest to yourself. How many times did you bathe in the sun this or last summer?

Let me guess.

If you are dark skinned, my guess is -- zero.
If you are white skinned there is the possibility of sun bathing.

In the past 10 years how many times have you purposely gone under the sun with the sole intent to make vitamin D? If you are black skinned whose attitude is "am too dark skinned for a sun bathe" you can still sun bathe until you feel the stinging pinch of the sun rays. This will take approximately 15 to 30 minutes. Black folks generally need more time in the intense Sun than Whites.

Can you start to see why the incidence of MS is now higher in Southern California black women than that of the other races? You should be able to see it. First, most black folks avoid the Sun and hardly eat foods plentiful in vitamin D. We do not go into the Sun as much as required. If we did, it will take intense sunlight and longer sunbathing times for our skin to start the necessary chemical reaction.

CHAPTER 3

Skin Color- Black or White

The color of your skin and one rule of thumb

People who have darker skin may also have trouble synthesizing vitamin D from the Sun if you live outside the equator. The pigment melanin, which is more prevalent in people with darker skin, reduces your body's ability to make vitamin D in response to sunlight exposure especially if you live in Europe and North American cities or countries.

For black skin people in equatorial Africa, they get the Sun rays straight. That is, they have the Suns' rays hitting the skin at an angle directly overhead. Out of the equator, you receive the rays at other angles not vertical. You receive your heat as oblique rays.

To make it simple, some rays are direct while others are oblique. Due to the curved surface of the Earth, some places receive more direct Sun rays than others. The direct Sun rays focus heat on an area. Less heat occurs where the rays are less direct-oblique. The people at the equator receive direct heat. Direct rays are called vertical because they come at you directly overhead.

Since the Earth is round, not all of the Sun rays strike the Earth in a vertical, or direct, manner. The less direct rays are called oblique rays. Oblique rays are spread out when they strike the Earth, and because of this they lose some of their heat.

Those at the equator has skin that is resistant to Sun rays. This makes it harder to convert Sun rays into vitamins. However, nature has a way of balancing things out. The black skin's resistance to the sun's rays is remedied by intense direct overhead sun rays. While the white skin does not have much of a resistance, it gets its vitamin D easier and faster. This is why a white skin requires lesser time while sunbathing in Central Park in New York.

Essentially, this means that people who have pale skin produce vitamin D more quickly than people with darker skin. So, places outside the equator suits pale skin well. Thus black skin outside the equator requires longer exposures to the sun's rays to get the type of benefit needed to avoid the consequences of vitamin D deficiency.

Skin-color typology is generally arranged into the following categories:

Type I - White; very fair; red or blond hair; blue eyes; freckles
Type II – White; fair; red or blond hair; blue, hazel, or green eyes
Type III – Cream white; fair; with any eye or hair color; very common
Type IV – Brown; typical Mediterranean Caucasian skin
Type V – Dark Brown; mid-eastern skin types
Type VI – Black

Thus, in the context of vitamin D production, if you have skin type I to III, you will produce vitamin D quicker than if you have the skin type IV to VI.

A good rule of thumb is to get half the Sun exposure it takes for your skin to turn pink to get your recommended amount of vitamin D. After you have exposed your skin for enough time, cover up with clothing and go back into the shade.

A dark-skinned African in North America might need 10 times or more sun exposure than a lighter-skinned person in North America to produce the same amount of vitamin D. Accept that as a rule of thumb when trying to bathe in the sun to get natural vitamin D.

CHAPTER 4

Photosynthesis of the skin

Now, can you imagine a plant not photosynthesizing? It turns yellow and dies. Humans not bathing in the Sun most often would not have enough of the sunshine vitamin and thus will develop sicknesses their parents never had.

How often have you been told that sunscreen reduces your ability to make vitamin D? Perhaps, you have never been told that. Sunscreen has been promoted as the remedy for avoidance of cancer while under the Sun—a must for preventing wrinkles and cancer. Hardly do you hear the part that says sunscreen reduces your skin's ability to make vitamin D by 90 to 99 percent and none at all --- depending on the level of SPF thoroughness of application.

In United States and environments like North America, it is even harder to catch the right rays without the sunscreen. Adding the sunscreen amounts to sitting under a dark cloud that allows no sun rays. Even at that, the sunlight you will most likely get on a daily basis, in the early mornings and late afternoons, is too weak to generate enough of this required vitamin.

Meanwhile, air pollution can filter out some of the UVB rays, so less of them are able to reach your skin at any time of the day.

The question is: How much sun is enough to get your daily dose of vitamin D? Is taking a vitamin D supplement sufficient?

The answer to this question is supposed to not apply to black Africans in the equator, but there are the rich ones whose daily pattern of behavior is to avoid the Sun. They go from air-conditioned rooms to air-conditioned cars and to air-conditioned offices and back to air-conditioned homes. This is the same pattern of life for many in the temperate zones during the summer.

Answer this question like this. How many hours did your father or grandfather spend in the farms while in the open Sun tilling the soil? The simple answer is -all afternoons and evenings--- minus a few resting hours. They had and still have -- a custom of going to the farm, so early in the morning (when the cock crows), so that by noon they are ready to take a break. Once the Sun tilts, they were back to work until sunset. For all that time, it is a whole lot of Vitamin D intake.

A good approach for researchers to take while considering research undertakings should be to measure the vitamin D level in the systems of such farmers. That will be an optimal way to determine the optimal level for vitamin D. Any other approach will be guesswork.

In all likelihood, these farmers are very likely to be very dark skinned. The darker you are, the longer it takes to make vitamin D. This must be one the variables if some researches are to be conducted. Leaving out this variable will obfuscate the results for peoples of dark skin everywhere in the world-- equatorial or temperate zones.

Most, if not all of the statistics obtainable on vitamin are results of studies of white people. So, if a report recommends 15 minutes of sun bathing for white skin, obviously the dark skin needs more. However, bear in mind that black skin can also get sun burn. Black skin comes in various degrees of melanin. Lots of black folks have the impression that they cannot be sun burned. Black folks in equatorial zones in Africa understands when to get in and out of the Sun. They know better not to be in the Sun from noon to about 2pm.

Seasons and the vitamin D levels:

Temperate zone's vitamin D levels vary throughout the year. However, it peaks in the month of August and receding around February. Levels of vitamin D in your body is very important to your health.

In one study, researchers analyzed genetic data from over 140,000 people of European descent in Europe and North America. The study found that for each 10 percent increase in vitamin D levels, there was an 8 percent decrease in the risk of developing high blood pressure otherwise known too as hypertension. This is just one in the many reasons why you should know the level of this vitamin in your system.

Generally, vitamin D levels have always been at its lowest during the winter months. The summer months are the bonanza months, when the Earth rotates and the angle of the Sun hits the atmosphere at an optimized angle for vitamin D production because more UVB reaches the places far away from the equator.

However, you must be in the Sun in those bonanza months to participate and enjoy the free, natural and organic source for vitamin D in order to attain your optimal levels. Even if you are in the equator areas of the earth, shielding yourself from the Sun rays will make you suffer the same fate as those in Europe and North America.

Have you observed that many African rich men living in equatorial Africa are beginning to acquire some foreign diseases at an alarming rate? Diseases like dementia, heart problems, broken hip bone, weak bones and cancer? Yes- cancer. That was not one of the big killers. It used to be malaria.

Most of the rich do not go under the Sun in Africa. They leave their air-conditioned houses for their air-conditioned cars and into the air-conditioned offices. They are likely not taking vitamin D supplements just like their fellow black folks in USA, Australia or England. How many times have you heard a black skinned fellow say out loud "I am not going under the Sun because I do not want to get darker?"

Now, you can appreciate that.

A 2000 study reported in the *Archives of Internal Medicine* has it that 77 percent of Americans are vitamin-D deficient.   OK. Let us digest that percentage. 77 percent. That simply means that for every four Americans, more than three are walking about not knowing that they are exposed to the potential of developing heart, cancer, multiple sclerosis and other problems.

According to the Centers for Disease Control (CDC), at least 31% of Blacks (cold weather blacks) are vitamin D deficient. Low levels of vitamin D are linked to lung disease, high blood pressure, sleep problems, depression, cancers, and diabetes to name a few. Research is finding that our sunlight needs are possibly not being met since we use sunscreen and are indoors more than necessary.

Numerous studies have shown vitamin D's crucial role in strengthening bones, fighting depression, and boosting immunity, but now, after decades of research and thousands of studies, experts may have finally proven that missing out on that one little letter d could be a major factor in pushing the number on your scale of bad diseases higher and higher.

Recent studies are drawing the conclusions that the recommended vitamin D daily intake levels are low- very low. Current guideline for vitamin D levels are too low because it took into account what was only needed for bone health.

Such guidelines leaves us susceptible to cancer and many other chronic diseases. What about our cardiovascular health?

Recently, the *Endocrine Society* took a bold step and created a new guideline based on overall optimal health requirements. This definitely is a way forward. Remember, those who live in the equator where their everyday activities in the Sun results in vitamin D production, have no need for debates on the dosage or guidelines.

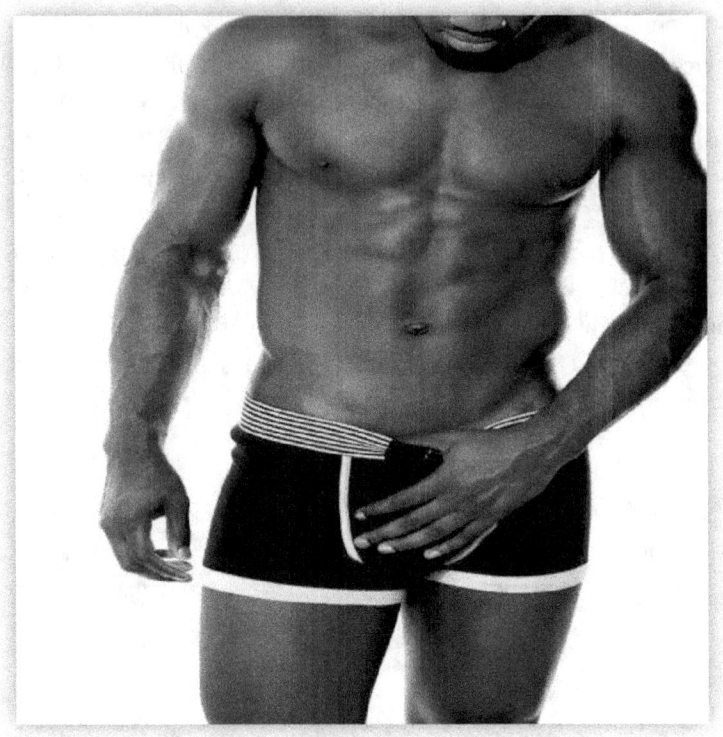

100% melanin from the sunshine vitamin

Nature, has taken care of dosage levels for blacks who bathe in the sun especially Africans in the equator.

Thus the *Endocrine Society* considered blood levels of vitamin D below:

20 ng/mL to be outright deficient,
21-29 ng/mL to be insufficient, and
30-100 ng/mL to be sufficient for achieving optimal health.

If you are deficient, you must bring it to optimal levels. In order to raise your vitamin D levels into the optimal levels around the weeks and months and year round, the *Endocrine Society* has recommended the following daily intake levels of vitamin D:

Babies under one-year-old: 400-1,000 IU/day
Children one - 18 years old: 600-1,000 IU/day
Adults: 1500-2000 IU/day

Some studies have rejected the above recommendations insisting that they are insufficient and therefore inadequate. And even at that, it is a level you cannot attain by diet only.

It is almost impossible to get these amounts through food alone.

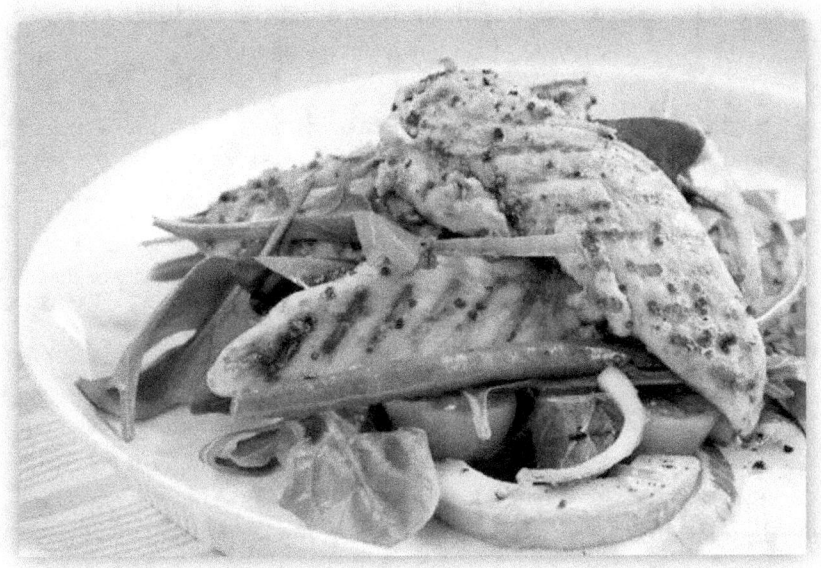

Sunbathing

Some recent studies in the U.S. have estimated that with food alone, women get fewer than 210 IU/day, men get less than 320 IU/day and children get less than 250 IU/day of vitamin D. That is sufficiently insufficient.

The right and sensible thing to do and rightly so, is to correct these gaps through supplementation.

The current upper limits for most children and adults range from 4,000 IU/day (*Institute of Medicine*) to 10,000 IU/day for adults (*Endocrine Society*). Never forget that the best way to be sufficient in vitamin D is a sensible Sun exposure for optimal health. The reason is this: you do not have to argue what the dosage should be. Africans in the equatorial do not have much of the dosage argument.

A container of vitamin D gels you can pick up from a supplement store is likely to read:

"Take 1 soft gel daily with a meal" and in a corner it will suggest that you pick your strength (incremental dosage) like this:

Regular: Active adults and children who consume a moderate amount of fish weekly

Double: Adults who do not exercise regularly or eat fish several times a week or may have some cardiovascular problems

Triple: Sedentary individuals who do not consume fish on a weekly basis or are concerned with high blood pressure.

(Regular = 1 gel is 2000 IU) so Triple = 6000 IU

Unfortunately, some of the latest research results confirm that many Americans and Canadians are outright deficient of this vitamin. It gets worse during the winter when our levels may drop as much as 50 percent and plunging deep into the "established" deficiency territory. The good news is that we now have some information, thus we can avoid unhealthy "D-efficient" levels with correct supplementation and, where possible, sunlight exposure in those winter days when the sun rays appears.

CHAPTER 5

Bleached Skin

Bleaching is the removal of the melanin. When the melanin is taken out, it exposes the white skin. What do you think is wrong with this picture? Why would anyone want to remove their natural skin? Simply put, it is due to ignorance, lack of information and/ or brainwashed.

Bleached skin is attainable for black people with whitening creams while not-so- white-skin is attainable for white skin by tanning. When you bleach, you expose yourself to all the diseases of the white skinned people. It is a double whammy. Cancer. Multiple sclerosis. Broken bones. Aging. You take your pick.

One more thing- when persons with bleached skin sweat a little, they stink up the space they are in.

Can you imagine a bleached skin under the Sun rays at the equator? If only the skin bleachers knew better. These lightening cream manufacturers are making lots of money on the ignorance of uninformed black people. They are at the same time getting users of lightening creams sick. Tell me about it—it is like paying the manufacturers to get cancer, MS, osteoporosis etc.

In some places in the equator, old men and women who perhaps have never seen a dentist, all their lives, still have their complete natural teeth intact. They hardly complain of broken bones or hips. Of course these are the old men in equatorial zones. They are strong and with their faculties intact. Dementia is rare among the old in the equator.

You can now see why in Africa, old people are hardly quarantined in old peoples home. This is because the chances for Alzheimer's is very low. *Alzheimer's* means the most common form of dementia, a general term for memory loss and other intellectual abilities serious enough to interfere with your daily life. According to available statistics, Alzheimer's disease accounts for 60 to 80 percent of dementia cases.

Obviously, we did not understand the power of vitamin D in a long time. We also did not understand the sun rays in a long time too. And seriously, the Africans had no need for such vitamin D knowledge then.

By the equator, black folks readily take the synthesis process of Sun and skin for vitamin D for granted and rightly so. You just do not think about that process because as soon as you step outside the house and the sunbathing starts, the process turns on.

So, most if not all blacks carry the mentality for taking the Sun for granted onto other continents when they emigrate. If you are a black person who lives or migrated to cold countries, your attitude is likely that of equatorial Africans.

You fall into that trap.

You forget about vitamin D. Have you considered the impact of insufficient vitamin D to your system? Do you take vitamin D supplements? If you never thought about it, think about it now and explain it to your neighbors near and far.

There is one thing black folks should never forget. That there is a reason they evolved to be black. Black skin was programmed to be black by nature. And some are unwittingly de-programming nature.

Nature does not play tricks. Nature must not be toyed with just for fun and when you want to toy with nature you better understand what the outcomes are. In this vitamin D discussion, some black folks are unknowingly toying with nature and there are consequences.

One of the consequences is multiple sclerosis. Multiple sclerosis (MS), also known as disseminated sclerosis is a demyelinating disease in which the insulating covers of nerve cells in the brain and spinal cord are damaged. Such damage can disrupt the ability of parts of the nervous system to communicate.

It is also known that higher levels of the hormone melatonin are linked to a lower incidence of multiple sclerosis (MS) flare-ups during the cold months of fall and winter.

When Africans were taken/emigrated from Africa, the skin type no longer fits the new cold climate. The less direct Sun rays of the new environment were not naturally suitable to a black skin. But they had no choice. The dark skin is designed to handle much more powerful Sun exposures that are much more intense. The sunlight in United States is not as intense as the equatorial sunlight neither are they as frequent UV-B rays.

The result is that the black skin-type overprotects the skin and not allowing it to produce enough vitamin D outside the equatorial zone. To make matters worse, African-Americans run away from the sun too. When white folks, vacation in Jamaica, Antigua or Santa Domingo--- one of the reasons is to sunbathe. When black folks vacation in these same places, care is taken to hide from the Sun.

This is why the majority of immigrants and people of African descent are vitamin D deficient in geographical locations where the sun rays are not as intense.

Milk is not enough weapon/food to protect and provide sufficient vitamin D for the black skin nor for the white skin for that matter.

Studies show that African-Americans and others with dark skin tend to be deficient in vitamin D.

Old people, black, overweight and obese tend to suffer the same faith. The reason is simple. Black folks outside Africa do not get their daily dose of vitamin D from the Sun, neither do they take supplements of vitamin D to make up the deficiency.

CHAPTER 6

Vitamin D and how it works

C an you think photosynthesis? Photosynthesis of the skin that is. When you sunbathe, skin photosynthesis takes effect. It works similarly like plant's photosynthesis that we learned in elementary school.

Not participating in this human photosynthesis is akin to sentencing self to a short life longevity. You notice that that tree that your great, great, great, great father climbed is the tree that you too climbed. The trees has a quality of senescence-aging so slowly that it is un-noticed.

Well, the Sun helps us to do that too. Hormone manufactured as a result from sunbathing helps you age with dignity and in good health. It elevates your level of senescence. Try to research aging in all the skin colors. Choose which skin color you would love to age as and keep that result to yourself.

Photosynthesis is the process by which green plants and certain other organisms transform light energy into chemical energy. During photosynthesis in green plants, that light energy is captured and used to convert H_2O (water), CO_2 (carbon dioxide), and minerals into O_2 (oxygen) and energy-rich organic compounds.

It is similar for humans when we are in the Sun sun-bathing. There are a few things that evolution/creation left to you to decide on.

Evolution made it possible for you to feel and recognize when to use the latrine/bathroom. Creation gave you the ability to sense when you are hungry. You can feel thirst and recognize it. There are however, things nature did not give you, and that is the ability to do it on your own-by yourself.

Nature did not give you the ability to control your sequence of breathing. If you had that ability, you will die while sleeping. There are activities that nature programmed to work by itself.

Nature programmed the skin to make vitamin D for the body. This is the one vitamin the body is programmed to make for self. Vitamin D is that important. It is so important, nature gave you that opportunity to evolve, to regulate and to adapt how you synthesize it, so that you do not come close to have the opportunity or carelessness to mess it up so very fast. After a while, you do mess it up though—all by yourself.

All you have to do, is go about your business in the Sun and your skin begins to synthesize the rays of the sun and does its human type photosynthesis.

And that simple task of sunbathing, most people, have not done well. They will mess it up. Many black folks are messing it up so badly, they have become so vitamin D deficient.

If you are one of the black persons outside the equator, you most likely have messed up. Are you one of the ones who messed up? Prove them wrong. Next time you see your doctor, request a vitamin D optimal level check.

Some white folks messed up but are recovering. Plants, especially those plants we keep at our homes- the plant that are vines, love the sun. No matter how dark a place you put them, they will grow towards the sunlight provided there are occasional light to that room. They just do it. The sunlight is so important for their survival. This process is called phototropism. You see, plants seek the light. And some black folks run from it.

Phototropism is the growth of plants, etc., in response to a light stimulus. It is mostly observed in plants but can occur in other organisms such as fungi. Plants' cells that are farthest from the light have a chemical called auxin that reacts when phototropism occurs.

This causes the plant to have elongated cells on the far side from the light. Growth towards a light source is called positive phototropism. Growth away from light is called negative phototropism.

In plants, it is mostly positive phototropism. Black skin has positive phototropism.

Like the human skin, plants rearrange their chloroplasts in the leaves so as to maximize photosynthetic energy and promote growth. Think of what happens to a plant without access to the sun?

Can you imagine the destiny of a plant that does not do this? It gets yellow, stunted and finally dies in a short period of time. One of my pet peeves is getting into a doctor's office and observe dead plants. If a doctor can't keep plants alive, he has no business in my body. Can you make that your pet peeve too?

The answers to those questions just about sums up reasons for majority of the deadly diseases we face when we have vitamin D deficiency.

Think of yourself as a tree in the forest. You have to grow taller so as to get all the sunlight or else other trees will suck up the sunlight. Then you get stunted in growth and not meet your potential. You would have a hell of a life. Vitamin D is as important to your body as oil is important to all countries or car production is important to German economy.

You should know how it works

Vitamin D is either absorbed by dietary intake or manufactured when epidermal 7-dehydrocholesterol converts UVB rays in the range of 290 nm to 310 nm hitting the skin into pre-vitamin D_3.

A thermal reaction causes pre-vitamin D_3 to convert into vitamin D_3, also named cholecalciferol, within the epidermis. What is more thermal than the Sun?

Vitamin D_3 is transported via vitamin D binding proteins to the liver, where it metabolizes into 25(OH) D, also named Calcifediol-a pre-hormone, the inert form of vitamin D.

Tightly regulated by parathyroid hormone, 25(OH) D converts to the active hormonal form of vitamin D, in the kidneys and other extra-renal tissues.
Other chemical reactions take place where the hormone binds to vitamin D receptors to regulate cellular function in several tissues located in the body, including brain neurons.

Simply put and in a layman's speak, this means that you burn off bad cholesterol and make good cholesterol at a faster rate.
Just think of all those stored bad cholesterol as a time bomb. How does burning off bad cholesterol sound to your ears? Lower bad cholesterol and increase in good cholesterol means extermination of many bad sicknesses.

CHAPTER 7

Deficiency of Vitamin D and the Implications

There are some findings in published articles using data from the Nurses' Health Study (NHS) database that suggests that there is an increased incidence of colon and breast cancer in postmenopausal women who have low vitamin D levels.

There are other conclusions from analysis of two studies. One found that women with serum 25(OH) D levels of more than 52 ng/ml had a 50% lower risk of breast cancer compared to women with levels less than 10 ng/ml.

In one review of colon cancer risk associated with vitamin D, it was found that higher UVB exposure and dietary supplement intake of vitamin D has an inverse relationship with the incidence of colon cancer.

Yet in another study it was found that the risk of developing autoimmune disease such as multiple sclerosis (MS), rheumatoid arthritis or type 1 diabetes is reduced in persons with adequate levels of vitamin D.

In an epidemiologic study it was found that where confounders such as UVB exposure and diet were not controlled, children who consumed 2000 IU of vitamin D daily during their first year of life had 80% less risk of developing type I diabetes compared to those who took less than this amount. Also in women, the risk of developing MS was reduced by 40% for those who consumed 400 IU of vitamin D daily. Remember, the dosage recommendation has been doubled or tripled.

In another follow-up study, for every 20 ng/mL increase in serum 25(OH) D among some white participants, the risk of developing MS was reduced by over 40%.

Benefits of Vitamin D

There are many benefits of vitamin D. Vitamin D deficiency is very harmful. Vitamin D has joined other vitamins like C and E as superstar vitamins.

Perhaps, we could say that vitamin C and E joined Vitamin D.

Vitamin D is good for your bones because it helps the absorption of calcium.

Optimal levels of vitamin D keeps increased risk of type 1 diabetes at bay.

Lower levels of this vitamin can lead to muscle and bone pain.

Optimal levels of vitamin D helps reduce the risk of cancers of the breasts.

Optimal levels of vitamin D helps reduce the risk of colon cancer.

Optimal levels of vitamin D reduces the risk of cancers of the prostate, ovaries and esophagus.

Optimal levels of vitamin D reduces' risks to the lymphatic system.

Optimal levels helps to regulate your immune system.

Vitamin D is one of the most potent inhibitors of cancer cell growth.

Vitamin D stimulates your pancreas to make insulin.

Optimal levels of vitamin D helps to normalize your blood pressure.

Optimal vitamin D lowers your chances of heart attacks.

Optimal levels of vitamin D reduces the chances of developing rheumatoid arthritis.

Optimal levels of vitamin D lowers your chances of multiple sclerosis (MS)

Optimal levels of vitamin D is good for healthy teeth.

Vitamin D is so important it plays a role in the determination of your life-time health at time of birth. There is a study from Cambridge University that found that the season in which you were born can influence how healthy you end up becoming as an adult.

Out of the equator, it can then be logically assumed that the "healthiest" birth months would be June, July and August. These are the summer months when the sun is very intense in Europe and America and all the non-equator zones. The Cambridge University study concluded too that the healthiest months were the summer months.

What then do you think of the healthiest birth months of countries in the equator following conclusions per the Cambridge study? The intensity of the sun in the equator is year round.

The study suggests that women who were born in the summer are more likely to be healthy adults. This new research was published in the journal *Heliyon*. The authors of the study, which involved half million people in the UK, suggests that more sunlight is readily available in the summer, therefore the effect is higher vitamin D exposure - in the second trimester of pregnancy. Though the study suggests this could explain the effect, they also cautioned that more research is needed.

The study suggests that birth month affects birth weight and other parameters. The mothers' sunlight exposure suggests when the girl starts puberty. Both birth weight and start of puberty have an impact on overall health in women as adults.

It will be necessary to recall that the researchers behind this new study from Cambridge University, UK, looked at whether birth month had an effect on birth weight, the start of puberty, and adult height. They concluded that children who were born in the months of June, July and August were approximately heavier at birth. They were also taller as adults and had an onset of puberty slightly later than those born in months other than June, July and August.

What do you take from the above study? Simply this: If you live in places outside the equator, planning and timing when your baby is due so as to fall into the summer months is advisable. However, you must take advantage of the Sun so as to avail yourself all the sunshine vitamin you can optimally get.

How does this apply in the equator regions? All you do is make sure that when and if pregnant, you do not remove yourself from the Sun by staying all day in an air conditioned room, air conditioned tinted car and air conditioned, sun blocking blinds office. Make time to enjoy the Sun. The Sun gives healthy life. It gives it abundantly.

Researchers believe that the differences in healthy babies and healthy adults could be traced to how much sunlight the mother got during pregnancy. To not have optimal sunlight exposure is like consciously exposing yourself to sickness instead of sun exposure.

CHAPTER 8

How To Get vitamin D

Specifically for Black man and woman:

Africans living outside of the equator and resident in places like Canada, Northern United States, Europe etc. are 25 percent more likely to contract and die from cancer than whites. There are plenty reasons. At earlier times it so easy to blame most sicknesses afflicting black folks in America to lower socio-economic status and little or no access to health care. Sometimes, the diagnosis of such illnesses are not done at the early stages.

However these aforementioned factors cannot fully explain the extent of disparities in survival for whites and blacks in America for the most common cancers and other sicknesses identified with vitamin D deficiency.

We now know that most detailed researches point the finger at a seemingly obvious but overlooked culprit: the Sun.

By now, you too, must have come to a conclusion that Vitamin D deficiency is common among African-Americans. This is because African-Americans shy away from sun rays. Some, even, buy creams to lighten up.

This lightening up behavior is occurring all over the globe where black people are resident. And did you know that the deficiency in vitamin D causes greater susceptibility to illnesses that are more ubiquitous in African-American and other black immigrants than among other ethnic groups?

Is any skin color, better than the other?
Is African-American skin color healthier
than the Caucasian skin color?

Before we answer the above question let us get some facts.

Let us establish one truth. Black people thrives better in the equator. White people are at their best health out of the equator. If the black race suddenly find themselves out of the equator, it is trouble. You may trick nature all you want but nature can get back at you for your treacherous behaviors.

So the answer to the question is relative because African (sub-Saharan) skin is an evolved skin perfected to life in the equator. For Africans in the equator they have nothing to worry about as far as they go outside under the rays of the Sun. For all other Africans not in the equator-African Americans, black immigrants in Europe, Russia etc., the specialty and efficiency of the black skin to make vitamin D through intense sun rays is lost.

This is because the black skin has more melanin. The more the melanin the need for intense sunlight increases. With a cold weather and not so intense sun in places like Northern America, the black skin's need can be met only if you get informed about the how. Thus, black folks in these regions are at a disadvantage. Sometimes, they forget or refuse to go under the intense sun in the summer. And it gets worse in the winter.

Meanwhile, the Caucasian or white skin is without melanin. It is an adaptation for life outside of the equatorial regions where the sun is significantly weaker than near the equator.

Because the white skin lacks melanin, it can quickly make vitamin D faster under a not so intense sunlight exposure. In these climates, the skin with melanin is at a disadvantage. Like the dark skin in the equator, white skin can adapt. So much so, that it changes hue to varying levels of sunlight exposure for the winter, fall, spring and summer. Thus, the white skin can synthesize vitamin D from less intense sunlight than that of the tropics. White skin is best suited for a temperate climate where sun exposure changes seasonally. In the equator, the white skin just cannot take the intense sun rays. If you try, you will scald badly in no time.

To therefore answer the question who is "healthier" then depends on where you live and your color. The white skin would suffer dire consequences in Africa (equator). The white skin offers low protection from the excess UV rays from sun exposure inside the equator. Therefore in the equator the black skin is healthier.

On the other hand, black skin is at a real disadvantage in temperate climes. It is worth repeating to all the African-Americans and African im-migrants in cold climes that black skin is very inefficient at synthesizing vita-min D from low intensity sunlight. The white skin is healthier in temperate climates. The black skin is not healthy in temperate climates and the truth is that most blacks do not know this. This is the simple reason many black folks get a result of vitamin D deficiency in temperate climates. It is not so in equatorial climes. If you are reading this and you are black, do somebody a favor and pass the information on. You could be the one that saves them from various cancers and other bad sicknesses.

It is a good practice to therefore supplement your diet with vitamin D while living in the northern latitudes especially if you are the type that runs from the Sun. Milk with fortified vitamin D is not sufficient. Lots of black folks are lactose intolerant anyway. To not supplement with vitamin D is therefore a double whammy. At this juncture you may wish to refresh your mind with the dangers of vitamin D deficiency.

Your number one source of vitamin D is the Sun. It is natural. It is or-ganic. This is the best source of this vitamin for black people. It has always been. Black skin is black for a reason. The Sun made black skin and it black skin manages intense sun rays much better than any other skin. Black skin is perhaps the end result of skin photosynthesis.

Though we can get vitamin D from foods and supplements, the Sun rays is black skin's longevity and health life line. Our ancestors knew this better even before science found the little it understands today. This is the one and only vitamin that nature allows you to make for yourself. Your ability to make and manage this function determines your health, longevity and quality of life. Your ability to sunbathe and make vitamin D determines your life de-void of multiple sclerosis (MS), broken bones, toothless mouth, high blood pressure, heart attack and especially cancer. We could go on and on about why you must not mess up this function but lots of people especially black people do mess this up.

There are a few black folks who do not mess this up in North America. Picture this. You see a few young black men walking in the streets with their pants hanging below the buttocks. They swagger as if their trousers is about to fall. The attempt to hold it from falling gives that swagger walk. They have at the top a wife-beater t-shirt or better still shirtless as they walk in the intense summer Sun.

Older people see these young men and see their fashion sense. Some even propose laws to be passed to regulate how these young people dress. That is not what I see. I see young black folks who unwittingly are sunbathing and making a lot of vitamin D that will prevent the chances of getting cancer, high blood pressure, heart attacks, multiple sclerosis etc.

They are unwittingly prepping for healthier adult life. I hope older folks would have this kind of Sun exposure to the body. The more frequent the exposure the better.

CHAPTER 9

Duration of Sunbathing

t is advised to get more than 90 percent of our vitamin D through Sun exposure. In Africa, Africans go into the sun daily. They bathe in the sun as they go about their daily affairs. They do not have a choice unless you are very rich.

By bathing, I don't mean lying on the grass while facing the Sun. It means that while in the equator, you have the benefit of baking in the Sun while walking to a friend's house or walking across the street to go get lunch or while fishing or farming. In any of these outdoor activities you engage in, you expose yourself to the sunshine vitamin.

This could last as little as five minutes to as much as six hours. Their skin has evolved for the Sun rays. You cannot actually put a time on it because some individuals work outdoors from sunrise to sunset. Majority of Africans in the equator get their 100 percent requirement of vitamin D from the sun.

According to the national Institute of Health, sunbath lasting between five and 30 minutes of sun exposure to your unprotected body in the hours when the sun is intense two to three times every week is enough for your body to produce all of the D3 it needs. Intense sun rays are between the hours of 10 a.m. and 4 p.m.

The extent or duration to stay in the sun varies. It also depends on whether you are black or white and all the other "ninety-nine" skin colors in between. There are recommendations. Some recommendations vary from fifteen to thirty minutes a day, with at least thirty percent of the skin surface exposed. Some recommendations suggest the arms and facial areas be exposed while others suggest that you also need your legs exposed in order to synthesize enough for optimal health.

Depending on your latitude, altitude, pollution levels, cloud cover, and skin color, you may need more sun exposure to generate the amount necessary for optimal health.

If black immigrants must learn from their forefathers they must learn this. They must learn from the ancestors in the equator. The African-Americans must learn the narrative of how our forefathers took advantage of the sunshine vitamin while working under the Sun.

Farmers in equatorial Africa up to this day scantily cover themselves. This meant that all the body except the buttocks and frontal areas are exposed. Scantily covered body lets the body sweat and receive cool breeze easily. The women also wear very loose clothing that exposes the whole body except the chest and waist areas. Meanwhile they are in the farms from sun rise (usually 6 a.m.) to about 12 noon when the Sun gets really intense. They take a break from about 12 noon to about 2 pm when the Sun is scorching. However, there are places that the Sun is so intense, you need clothing to cover almost all parts of the body except the eyes. It has nothing to do with religion.

This is the same pattern for builders, fishermen, construction workers, etc. in good old days and continues to this day.

Even in their everyday fashion, clothing are usually designed so that much of the body is exposed to take advantage of the sunshine vitamin.

The amount of white skin you expose – if you wear clothing that covers most of your skin, you may be at risk for vitamin D deficiency. This also means that people who train indoors in the winter months may have to rely on their bodies' vitamin D stores, which further increases their risk for deficiency. Please understand also that cloudy weather can be a problem because lesser and not so intense Sun rays will reach the skin on such days. You can always supplement but ask your doctor.

CHAPTER 10

Sunscreens

have seen and observed a few black folks buy sunscreens in temperate zones. My feeling and urge was to ask them---why? I am wondering what the need is for a black person to buy sunscreen. Is it a waste of money and time? What is the benefit? Unless, you want to feel bourgeoisie, black skin has little or no need for sunscreens.

Sunscreen was manufactured for the use of white people. They did not have the black folks in mind while doing studies with white skin samples.

How does it work?

Sunscreen combines organic and some inorganic chemicals designed to filter the light from the Sun so that less of it reaches the deeper layers of the white skin. Like a screen door, some light penetrates the skin, but not as much as if the door was not present. The summary of it is that it reduces the intensity of Sun rays penetration.

Sunblock disperses or scatters the light away so that it does not reach the skin. Now, you can see why making vitamin D under this circumstance is hard. With a black skin, it's nearly impossible.

The particles that helps in reflecting the light in sunblock usually consist of zinc oxide or titanium oxide. Sunscreens are likely to include sunblock as part of their active ingredients.

It is easy to tell who was using a sunblock just by looking as the sunblock whited out the skin. Today, not all brands of modern sunblock are visible because the oxide particles are smaller, though you can find the traditional white zinc oxide.

That portion of the sunlight that is reflected away or blocked is the ultraviolet radiation. There are three regions/levels of ultraviolet light. The Sun is a source of the full spectrum of ultraviolet radiation which is commonly subdivided into UV-A, UV-B, and UV-C.

Ultraviolet light has shorter wavelengths than visible light. Although UV waves are invisible to the human eye, some insects, like the bumblebees, can see them. This is also similar to how a dog can hear the sound of a noise from a whistle just outside the hearing range of humans.

UV-A penetrates deeply into the skin and is responsible for causing cancer and premature skin aging.

UV-B is usually responsible for tanning and burning/scalding of white skin. A certain amount of shortwave ultraviolet radiation (UVB) must penetrate the outer skin layer in order for the body to produce vitamin D.

UV-C is usually and completely absorbed by the earth's atmosphere.

For black people, nature has done its work for their protection. Nature provides melanin. Melanin is normally located in the epidermis, or outer skin layer.

It is produced at the base of the epidermis by cells called melanocytes. These cells have photosensitive receptors that detect ultraviolet radiation from the sun and other sources.

They respond by producing melanin within a few hours of exposure. Nature has selected for people with black skin in tropical latitudes, especially where ultraviolet radiation from the sun is usually very intense.

The take from this is: the black is suited for intense sunlight. The black skin is not evolved to avoid the sun. If you are black and you are in the habit of avoiding the Sun, you are negating the intent of nature. The black skin needs the intense Sun to make its body's vitamin D needs.

Melanin acts as a protective biological shield against ultraviolet radiation. Therefore, it helps to prevent sunburn damage that could result in DNA changes that leads to several kinds of malignant skin cancers.

Melanoma in particular is a serious threat to life. In the United States for example, approximately 55,000 people acquire this very aggressive type skin cancer every year and nearly 10,000 of these die.

Those at highest risk are white folks. They have a 10 times higher risk than African Americans.

However, African Americans are beginning to fall prey to these aggressive type illnesses because they are avoiding the sunlight or they are not getting the right level of vitamin D. For African Americans, it is advisable to ask your doctor to do a vitamin D deficiency test a couple of times a year. African Americans' penchant to run away from the Sun negates the biology of melanin.

There are a few reasons people advance for applying sunscreen on their skin. Let us list a few.

1. To prevent scalding.
2. The ozone layer is depleting so I have to protect my skin.
3. Skin cancer is on the rise. Sunscreen would help prevent cancer.
4. It helps in the slowing down of wrinkled and premature aging skin.
5. It helps reduce the appearance of facial red veins and blotchiness.
6. It helps to prevent facial spots and skin discolorations.

Sunscreen can block vitamin D production. Using sunscreen is not actually recommended to protect your skin. Shades and clothing can do the same or better job. This is because sunscreen has not consistently been shown to prevent all types of skin cancers. The truth of the matter is that if you want your skin to absorb UVB rays that are necessary to synthesize vitamin D3, you just cannot wear sunscreen. There are studies that have found that sunscreens with sun protection factor (SPF) 8 or higher block the skin's ability to produce vitamin D from sunlight by as much as 95 percent.

What Does SPF Mean

SPF is the acronym for Sun Protection Factor (SPF). It is also a number that helps to determine how long you can sunbathe before getting a sunburn.

Sunburns and scalding are caused by UV-B radiation. SPF does not indicate protection from UV-A. The UV-A causes cancer and premature aging of the skin.

The skin has a natural SPF, partly determined by how much melanin your skin makes, or the degree of black the skin is. The SPF is therefore a multiplication factor. What this means is that if your white skin can withstand the sun for 30 minutes before getting sunburn, the use of an SPF of 10 would help you withstand the sunlight by ten times longer without burns. 10x 30 equals 300minutes.

Although the SPF only applies to UV-B, the labels of most products will indicate whether they offer broad spectrum protection. There usually should be some indication of whether or not they work against UV-A radiation. Remember the UV-C is entirely contained by the atmosphere. The particles in sunblock reflects or deflects UV-A and UV-B.

How Much Ultraviolet Radiation Is Filtered By Transparent Glass?

Glasses that are transparent to visible sunlight absorbs most of UV-B regions. UV-B is the wavelength range that can cause sunburn. Does this mean that the white skin cannot get sunburn while behind such glasses? Yes. It is true that the glasses protects you from getting a sunburn. It therefore means that making vitamin D too is harder for black skin or any skin for that matter since the glass absorbs most of the UV-B light. It is that region of the ultraviolet radiation you need to make the sunshine vitamin.

However, UV-A is much closer to the visible spectrum than UV-B. Approximately, 75% of UV-A pass through transparent glass. UV-A leads to DNA damage and genetic mutations that ultimately leads to cancer. Glass does not protect you from skin damage from the Sun as much of UV-A will pass through it.

CHAPTER 11

Foods That Contain Vitamin D

The Sun remains the best way to get vitamin D, however, there are foods that contain vitamin D and they are few.
Only a few foods contain vitamin D naturally.

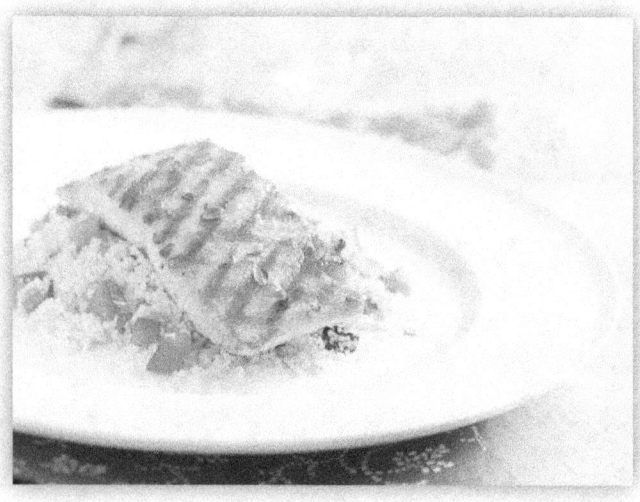

Fish

You can get Vitamin D from some fortified foods, as well as from many types of fish, some mushrooms, and egg yolk, but by far the best way to get enough Vitamin D is through Sun exposure of our skin.

See the photo below for foods containing vitamin D.

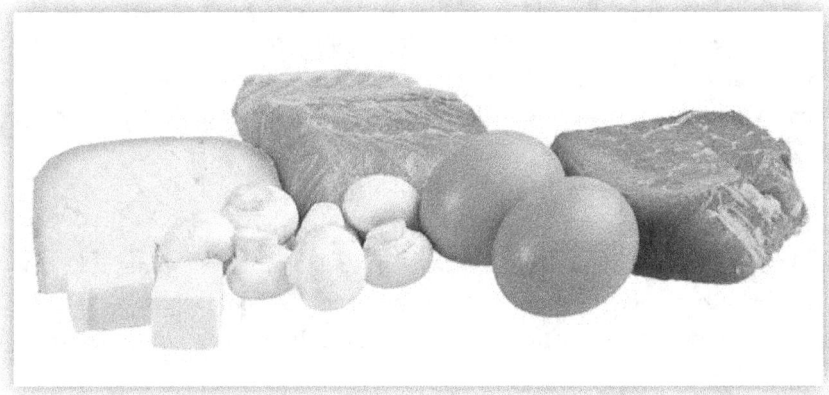

These fortified foods include oily fish (salmon and or mackerel), cod liver oil, irradiated mushrooms, and egg yolk.

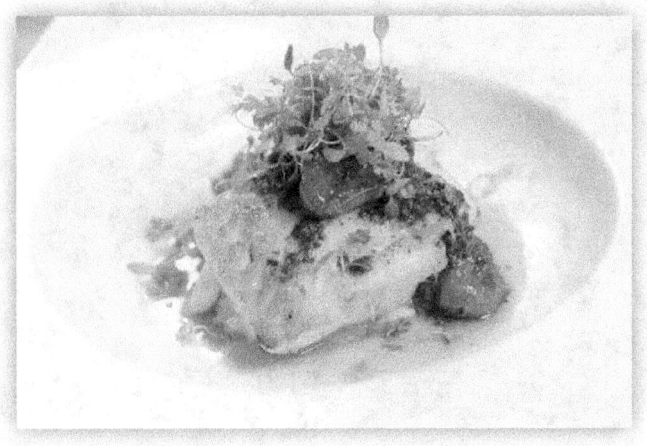

Foods fortified with vitamin D may include orange juice, milk, other juices, yogurt, cheese, cereal and breads. Getting your needed level of vitamin D in a temperate climate is usually difficult. Getting your daily optimal dose of vitamin D in the equator can be accomplished just by stepping outside for a few minutes and not even think about it.

Although the amounts of vitamin D vary, and several servings of the above mentioned foods need to be consumed so as to meet the minimum daily requirement of vitamin D. Of course common sense tells us that that would be mostly impossible. It is highly recommended to add dietary supplements.

Dietary supplements can contain either vitamin D_2 or vitamin D_3. My doctor recommended Vitamin D_3 which is thought to have greater efficacy in elevating serum 25-hydroxyvitamin D (25[OH] D) levels compared to vitamin D_2.

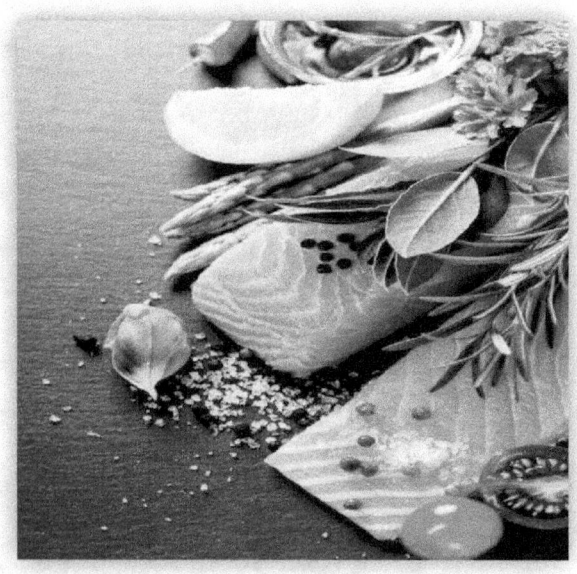

The dietary intake of vitamin D that is required to obtain optimal levels of serum vitamin D to maintain many body functions is still being debated by leading researchers. And it is a hot debate for white folks.

Such debates hardly exist in equatorial Africa. That is because it is not important for the inhabitants not because they are black but because they get the Sun in abundance and the black skin has determined what dosage it needs.

However, as soon as a black skin person emigrates to the white man's climate, your vitamin D intake becomes compounded and the hot studies raging on becomes even more important for you.

If you are black who emigrated out of the equator, you must pay close attention to the study because it cannot be any more important to a white skin than it is to the black skin. If anything, the black peoples in temperate zones are the ones that are always more likely to have vitamin D deficiency- a reason the study needs to be taken seriously. My hope is that enough black folks are included in the samples used in the studies.

Currently, the Institute of Medicine has established the adequate intakes (AI) of vitamin D at:

200 IU/day for adults up to 50 years of age
400 IU/day for adults aged 51 to 70 years and
600 IU/day for adults over 71 years of age.

However, a recent risk assessment of vitamin D revealed that these AIs are too low to maintain optimal vitamin D level and concluded that the safe upper limit of daily vitamin D adequate intake should be 10,000 IU/day.

There is a simple question for you. Rather than that study said this and this other study said that with regards to adequate AI, why not just go out in the Sun and sun bathe for a few minutes three times a week? Even in the winters, the Sun still shines every now and then.

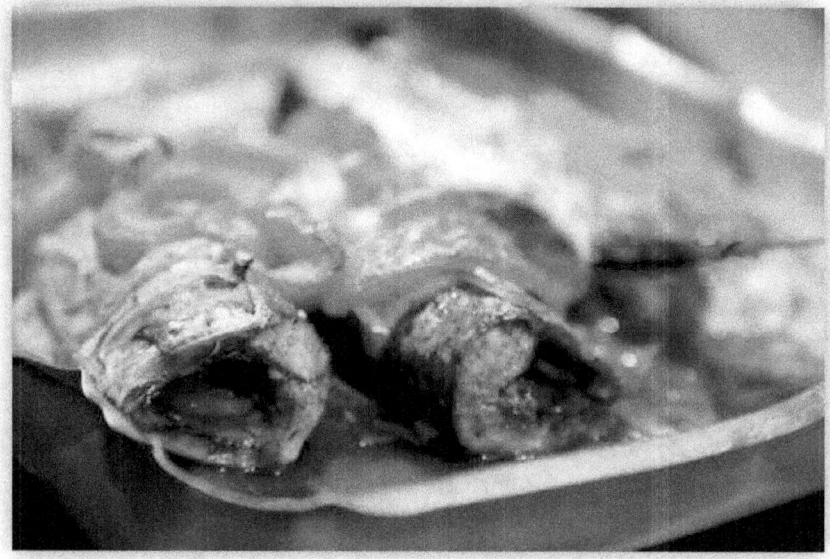

CHAPTER 12

More Benefits of Vitamin D

Your body naturally makes vitamin D when your skin is exposed to sunlight. The form of vitamin D that you get from the sun is called D3. It is also known as cholecalciferol which is derived from cholesterol.

The amount of vitamin D you get from exposing your bare skin to the Sun is dependent on several factors two of which are your skin color and intensity of the Sun.

Vitamin D is a necessary nutrient to preventing rickets. Today, vitamin D has become famous primarily for helping your body absorb calcium to enable strong bones.

In the past few years, there has been a number of research linking Vitamin D deficiency to a range of medical conditions such as osteoporosis, multiple sclerosis, heart disease, and the various different cancers. Other conditions include depression, high blood pressure, diabetes, seasonal affective disorder, migraines, rheumatoid arthritis, PCOS, influenza, prostate health, infertility and many others. As results of more studies are published, it is certain that other conditions will be discovered.

Vitamin D and control of temperament

Receptors in the brain need vitamin D to keep hunger and cravings at optimal levels. Vitamin D enables high levels of the mood-elevating chemical--- serotonin.

Vitamin D optimizes the body's ability to absorb other important weight-loss nutrients like calcium. If the body lacks calcium, it experiences up to a fivefold increase in the fatty acid synthase, an enzyme which helps to convert calories into fat.

In a 2009 study published in the *British Journal of Nutrition*, it was reported that obese women who were on a 15-week diet and who took 1,200 milligrams of calcium a day lost more weight than women who followed the diet without 1,200 milligrams of calcium.

What this means is that by allowing Vitamin D in your system your body stores less fat as it turns into an optimally fat burning efficient machine.

Scientists now know that vitamin D is the biochemical key that releases the most stubborn fat in your cells so our body can burn it off instead of storing such fat on the hips, buttocks, thighs, and stomach. If you are fat, chances are that you do not go under the Sun or perhaps not taking vitamin D supplements.

Sunscreen and Vitamin D

As already explained, many natural and conventional health care practitioners are concerned that the push to always wear sunscreen and avoid the sun at all costs has helped contribute to a lot of people having suboptimal vitamin D levels. This is why. The same sunscreen we are putting on to prevent skin cancer is also blocking our body's ability to make vitamin D.

Our bodies require UV light to make vitamin D, and sunscreens block out UV light. A sunscreen that has an SPF of 8 blocks your ability to synthesize vitamin D by approximately ninety three percent. An SPF of 15 blocks nearly ninety-nine percent of your ability to make Vitamin D.

How then do we reconcile this new information with the mantra of past years to always wear sunscreen to cover every exposed part of our body at all times we are in the sun?

Remember that available statistics has cancer rates higher than usual. So, the question is: why is it that despite sunscreen use, skin cancer rates are still high? You would think that the use of sunblock and sunscreen would have reduced the incidence of cancer.

So far we have seen results of many studies that lists the benefit of vitamin D as a cancer prohibiting agent.

So the debate that if Vitamin D is shown as a cancer-fighting hormone, what is the logic behind blocking its production through sunscreen? If we do that we are inadvertently making skin cancer rates worse.

On the other hand, there is a lot of evidence showing that sunscreen and sunblock reduce sunburns thereby preventing skin cancer. The benefit of sunscreen must not be lost especially for white folks.

Sunscreen makes life during the summer months bearable for those at the various beaches around the world especially for white skin peoples. Sunscreen makes it possible for white folks to enjoy in a bearable manner, the beautiful summer days without suffering burns and peels.

So what do we do? Find out in the next chapter.

CHAPTER 13

Conclusion

The way some people avoid the sunlight makes it seem like the sun is waging a constant war against our skin. We know that harmful UV radiation burns our skin. It damages our DNA and thus sow the seeds for melanoma.

However, the Sun is essential for our healthy development and our immune systems because Sun exposed skin produces vitamin D.

So, to really maximize the ability of the skin to make this vital vitamin and not get burned, there has to be a middle ground. As with lots of things, for example alcohol, moderation may be the best course of action. Like too much alcohol, too much Sun exposure, and the flip option of never having any sun exposure, are both proving to have unintended deadly consequences. We will make more specific recommendations later.

When it comes to staying healthy and looking great, it is very important to not be deficient in any vital vitamin. Vitamin D is no exception and definitely not the vitamin to be deficient in. Vitamin D is an important vitamin for the body for so many reasons. Vitamin D helps the body to functionally work better. For women in particular--black or white skinned, Vitamin D is important for you because it contributes to healthy looking beautiful skin.

Have you heard or touched the ebony black skin woman? It radiates and shines like it is reflecting the Sun. It is elastic and vibrant.

The fact is that the body makes vitamin D naturally. This function of the skin decreases as you start to age. Supplementation is therefore necessarily as we age. It is a good idea to discuss that with your doctor.

Unfortunately, since Vitamin D decreases naturally in the body as one ages, people who are not able to get an adequate amount of Vitamin D from the Sun might find that they are deficient in Vitamin D because they are not receiving it naturally from the environment. In cases such as this, a vitamin D supplement is highly recommended to keep a balanced skin tone overall.

A vitamin D supplement is needed to perfectly parallel the natural effects of the Sun. The benefits that vitamin D can afford your skin are many and varied. It could be in the reduction of acne, increase in the elasticity in the skin, decreasing the fine lines of wrinkles as well as dark spots. Vitamin D makes your skin glow and extremely radiant.

Recommendations:

- Go outside daily where possible for 15-30 minutes with minimal clothing exposing your arms and legs to the intense sun.
- If you intend to be under the intense sunlight for extend period put on a EWG approved sunscreen to avoid those chemicals that might make skin cancer worse.
- Take a daily vitamin D supplement on days you are not under the intense sunlight and especially during the winter months when intense sunlight is not readily available to boost what is naturally being made by our bodies.
- Have your vitamin D levels checked at least once or twice a year to know what our levels measure. Where possible, do this test during

the winter months. Be aware that Vitamin D can be toxic in large doses. It is advisable to know your levels before starting any high-dose supplementation.

- Discuss RDA with your doctor. The published RDA for Vitamin D is technically 200-400 IU a day. There is a dispute with that as research suggests that that number may be too low to maintain adequate Vitamin D levels. There is a difference between an RDA and Adequate Intake (AI).
- If you make a choice to supplement, choose the D3 form, not D2.
- If you are a black person living in a temperate climate, stop avoiding the sun. If you do, please supplement.
- If you are black in cold weather environment, you need to Sun expose the skin longer and regularly.

When it comes to vitamin D, like in real estate, it is location, location, location.

You are good if you are in the equator and you do not hide from the sun and do not supplement.

You are good if you are not in the equator but you expose your skin regularly to available sunlight or otherwise supplement.

Black and white people need to avoid the ignorance and lack of consensus within the medical and scientific research community regarding vitamin D's supplementation and/or sun exposure.

During this past summer, I spent a lot of time in a project that required I work outdoors. I was in group of eleven black and white folks of both sex. I noticed that most of them were avoiding the sun. While the white folks were genuinely avoiding the sun for fear of sunburn and peels, the black folks were avoiding the sun for fear of getting "darker". Ironic, isn't it?

It appears, at least to me, that regardless of a person's educational status, the vast majority of people are at best lukewarm in taking responsibility for their own health and wellbeing– and this can be whether we are talking about food, diet or vitamin supplementation. With regards to vitamin D and sun exposure, we find that many people are not properly informed—even those in the medical community.

People usually turn to their physicians for health care matters because they trust their physicians completely. But physicians are humans. They cannot know everything and sometimes they make mistakes. Sometimes, you need to help your doctor to help you by doing some reading on your own on what ails you. Information you gather through your research enables you to ask your doctor intelligent questions. It is based on what you tell your doctor that s/he proceeds to diagnose your ailments.

I am hoping that those physicians who understand the extreme importance of vitamin D to our health and wellbeing become more outspoken; and take an approach that educates their patients and thus the public.

While plants continue to use the sun through process of photosynthesis to be bountiful and disease free, my hope is for man to understand that man's own photosynthesis takes place too under the Sun not outside it.

Do not put your personal photosynthesis on hold. Unfortunately for some, it is on hold because scientists cannot agree on acceptable method(s) under which human photosynthesis can take place. It is that process used by plants and other organisms to convert light energy, normally from the Sun, into chemical energy that can be later released to fuel the organism's wellbeing.

Remember: Talk to your doctor about the safe use of supplements.

References

Online resources.

http://www.cdc.gov/cancer/skin/statistics/race.htm

http://www.neurology.org/content/80/19/1734.abstract

Other e-books
by Jay Parker

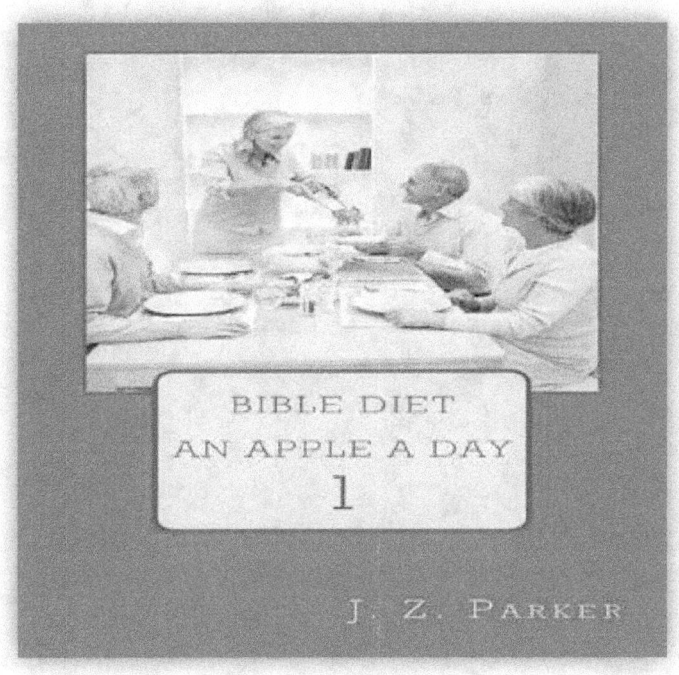

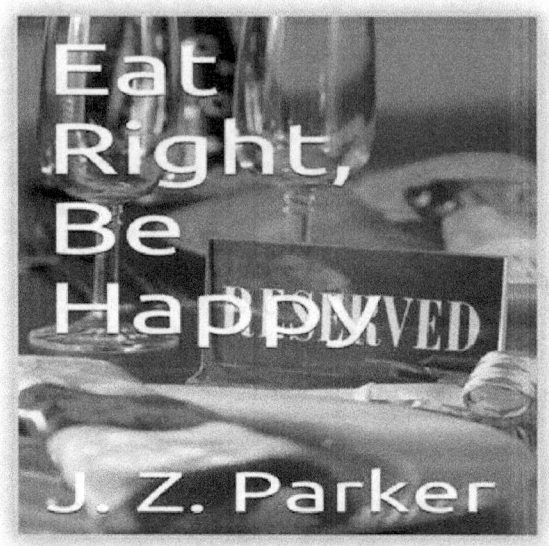

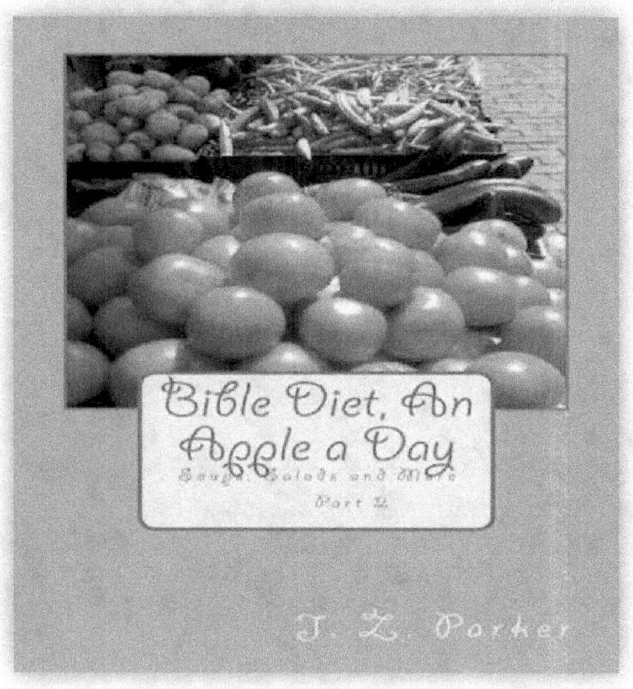

www.ingramcontent.com/pod-product-compliance
Lightning Source LLC
Chambersburg PA
CBHW071229280526
45787CB00002B/859